# IBOGA AND IBOGAINE

## An Overview

K M Schaeffer

**KMS Freelancing**

ISBN-13: ISBN: 9798395687098
Imprint: Independently published

Cover design by: Art Painter
Library of Congress Control Number: 2018675309
Printed in the United States of America

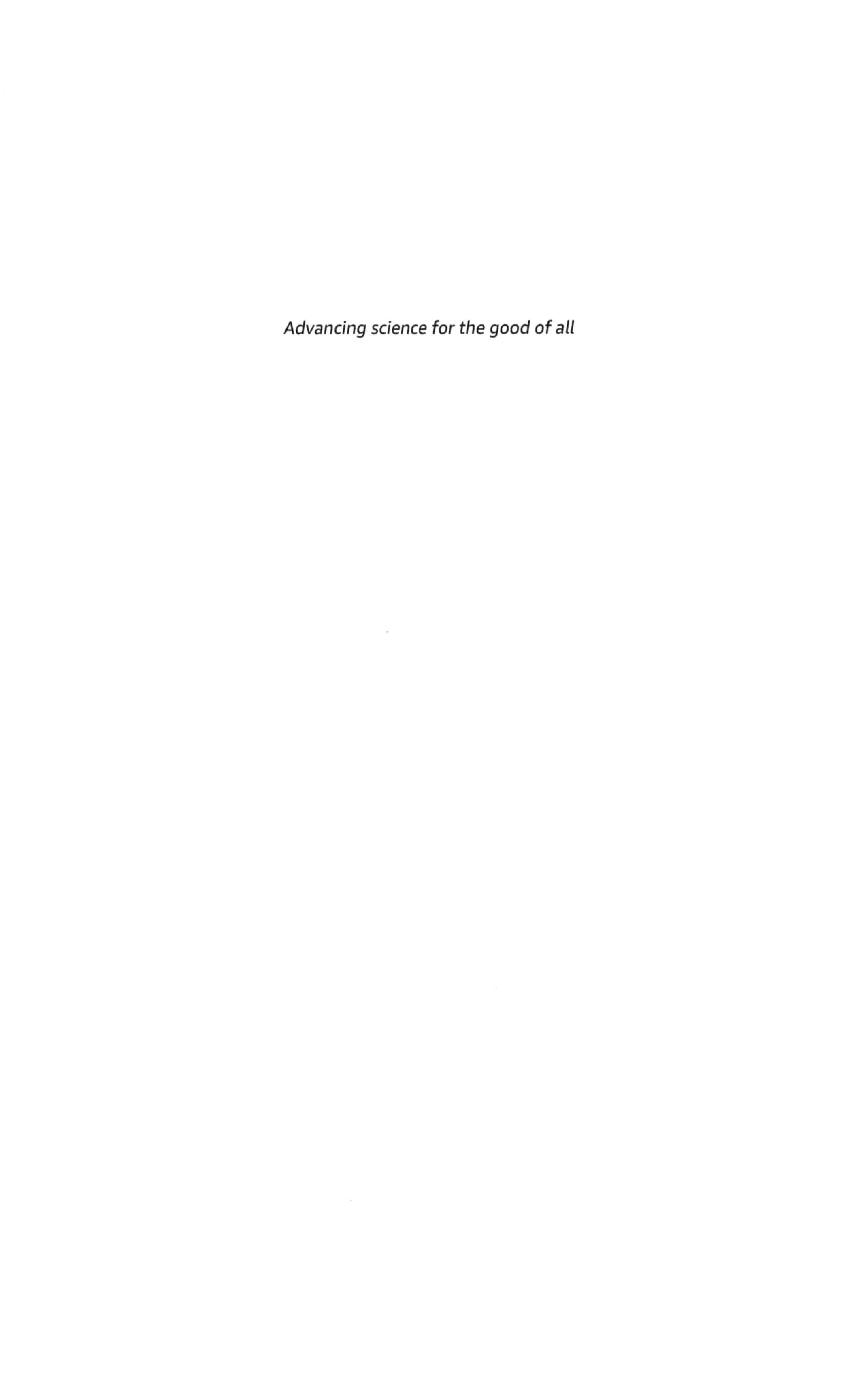

*Advancing science for the good of all*

# Iboga Ceremony
## By K M Schaeffer

The resurgence of a little known herb

The use of psychedelic plants for religious purposes is an ancient practice, and it is ubiquitous among many native cultures and often incorporates healing, magic, and teaching traditions.

The profound alterations in consciousness brought about by the use of psychedelics have served as a foundation for countless spiritual and religious systems. Examples of this can be found on every continent (with the exception of Antarctica) and in almost every culture.

Examples can be found all throughout the world. Take for exampleworldIf you look, in the tribes and people of the jungles of the Amazon, you'll find many there many cultures can be found that use ayahuasca and yopo (DMT and 5-MeO-DMT, respectively), movinge further north into Mesoamerica, and there is a great deal of evidence pointing to the the historical use of psilocybin-containing mushrooms. Traveling a bit further north into the Americas, and there are multiple native tribes that still use peyote (mescaline) in many of their ceremonies. Crossing the Atlantic into Eurasia, can also find the use of you historically another fungus, Amanita Muscaria, as well as henbane was used in many parts of eastern Europe and played a major role in lots of early Eurasian folkelore. Finally, head back in history to the cradle of humanity in Africa, and there is one plant that is used throught the Sehel reigionyou'll find the use of Iboga (Ibogaine), whose use that dates back centuries.

Out of all the traditional psychedelics, Iboga is one that stands out in two very distinct ways. First iIt was the only psychedelic to be prescribed for nonpsychiatric purposes, and secondly for a brief period and for the broad cascade of neurotransmitters Consuming it causes.are released. Between the 1930s and 1960s, ibogaine extract was sold to promote mental and physical stimulation, and was quite popular in France as Lambarène. Despite being identified by French explorers in 1889 with its primary active alkaloid, Ibogaine, being isolated in 1901 by Dybowski and Landrin (1), its activity went largely unknown. Recently, iboga has gained  attention from the broader scientific community as a powerful tool in the age of the opioid epidemic.

# WHAT IS IBOGA?

Iboga, scientifically known as Tabernanthe iboga, is a perennial shrub found in the rainforests in Equatorial Africa. It has dark green, narrow leaves on woody stems with clusters of white tubular flowers. These flowers create yellow-orange fruits. These fruits look very close to the average Chili pepper.

Like most plants, iboga creates a range of nitrogen-containing chemicals, referred to as alkaloids, designed to aid the plant's survival. Plants and animals commonly produce alkaloids that contain antibacterial, antifungal, and toxic compounds that help the organism's resilience.

Take, for example, the poison dart frog. It creates a mixture of highly toxic alkaloids, batrachotoxin, epibatidine, and histrionicotoxin, to name a few, that helps keep it from being predated by bigger animals. Sometimes, these toxic alkaloids can have a pretty unique effect on humans.

Iboga is a perfect example of a plant whose alkaloids exert not only a physiological response, such as pain relief or lowering a fever, but instead will create pronounced psychological effects ranging from a slight stimulation and mild pain relief with low doses to visionary experiences with higher doses. These high doses which are used in various ceremonies by multiple peoples including those people practicing Bwiti. The main alkaloids, Ibogaine, Noribogaine, Yohimbine, and a few others, comprise about 6% of the total plant material. Although this may seem like a tiny amount, they are responsible for the plant's powerful visionary effects. Ibogaine, one of the most active alkaloids, is responsible for causing quite strong visionary and introspective effects in people who consume either the plant whole or the extracted alkaloid.

# HISTORY OF IBOGA

The use of iboga is one of the oldest systems throughout the African Continent that has evolved into a spiritual discipline. One that is still practiced today. The practice is known as Bwiti. Bwiti is historically common among the Punu and Mitsogo peoples of Gabon and the Fang people of Cameroon. This spiritual practice focuses on the use of the psychedelic effects of the iboga plant, along with other ceremonial rituals, to promote radical spiritual growth, help to stabilize the community and family structure, fulfill religious requirements, and as a way of healing physical ailments.

In the words of the chief physician and a professor of Tropical Medicine in France, Bureau said, "Gabon is to Africa what Tibet is to Asia, the spiritual center of religious initiations."(9) As you can imagine, Bwiti became normalized and popularized in the region. People who are initiated "will see the Bwiti only twice. On the day of his initiation and the day of his death."

The first record of Iboga shows up in western literature in 1864 when Charles Eugène Aubry-Lecomte described it in his short essay on the plant poisons of West Africa after he returned from exploring the area. In his essay, he remarked (that iboga) "is only toxic in high doses and the fresh state. Taken in small quantities, it is an aphrodisiac and stimulant of the nervous system; warriors and hunters use it to stay awake during their night vigils" (3). Up to this point, all that was truly known about the plant is that it could provide mild stimulation and that at higher doses, it would cause ataxia, which is a difficulty in coordinating muscle motion that can make standing and walking almost impossible. The other thing that was known was and that high enough doses could have cardiotoxic effects. Aside from that, Iboga was seen as relatively unremarkable, and no further studies were done on it, or Ibogaine.

Even though ibogaine was first isolated and then synthesized in 1901, it took until the 1970s for any scientist to seriously investigate its pharmacodynamics. The study of pharmacodynamics looks at a compound's subjective and physical effects and the mechanism(s) of its action. One feature that is unique to Iboga, and therefore Ibogaine, is that it acts as an agonist on a wide range of neurotransmitters and their systems. This means that it binds to, or affects almost every neurotransmitter. While most drugs such as opioids only bind to one set of receptor, s, in this case, it binds to three sets of opioid receptors. ibogaine binds to or has an effect on seven different neurotransmitter systems.

None of this was known until fairly recently. It took until the late '80s,early '90s for the first scientific studies exploring the binding activity of ibogainethe drug to be conducted. As the story goes, Howard Lotsof, an American scientific researcher who would later go on to write the first studies on the anti-addictive properties of Ibogaine, stumbled across the use of ibogaine as a treatment for heroin addictions such as . Hhis own and those of his friends. This was when the research began in earnest, launching a new era into the study of Ibogaine.

As Lotsof states in a New York Times article from 2010, "while [my] interest in ibogaine may have started with this drug party, the unique effects of ibogaine became immediately evident in that it was not a substance conducive to such parties. There followed a period of six months of lay research, which provided a dose-related response study ranging from 1 mg/kg to 19 mg/kg of ibogaine in both the addict and non-addict human subjects." These experiences jumpstarted what he would call his "humanitarian mission," to help treat addicts.

By 1985 Howard Lotsof was off to the races. He began writing papers and taking out patents. His first was a U.S. Patent on a Rapid method for interrupting the narcotic addiction syndrome (6), followed by another just one year later in 1986 on a Rapid method for interrupting the cocaine and amphetamine addiction syndrome (7). Then in the coming years, he took out two more patents. One in 1989 for a Rapid method for attenuating the alcohol dependency syndrome (8) and the other in 1991 for a Rapid method for interrupting or attenuating the nicotine/ tobacco dependency syndrome (9).

# HOW DOES IBOGA WORK?

As mentioned before, unlike most psychoactive compounds that affect one or two neurotransmitters, Ibogaine affects most of the neurotransmitters in the brain. Like all classical psychedelics, such as LSD and psilocybin, ibogaine binds to the 5-HT2a receptor. It is widely accepted in the scientific community that stimulating this subset of the serotonin receptors is responsible for most of the hallucinogenic associated with most psychedelics. One thing that makes iboga and ibogaine so unique is that they also bind to several other receptors. It is also active at all three opiate receptors, the NMDA receptor, which affects glutamate, the nicotinic acetylcholine receptors, and the serotonin and dopamine transporter systems (8).

The main psychedelic effects can be attributed to two receptors. First, the 5-HT2a serotonin receptor, like most classical psychedelics. Secondly and quite unique to psychedelics, the kappa opioid receptor. While as unintuitive as it seems, this action of ibogaine at the kappa opioid receptor adds significantly to the plant's psychoactive properties. We know this because of another plant that is recognized for having strong hallucinogenic properties, Salvia Divinorum, known as salvia to most. Interestingly enough, salvia's psychedelic effects are entirely due to a chemical that is highly selective at the kappa opioid receptoragonist.

## *What is the Iboga (Ibogaine) experience like?*

Iboga and its isolate Ibogaine have been reported to be one of the more challenging compounds to work with. Physically, this is primarily due to the purge inducing effect, and the fact that the peak effects can last between 18 and 30 hours. After effects can linger for 24 to 72 hours.

Within the first hour or two of taking ibogaine, people report starting to feel a numbing of the skin, often accompanied by an auditory buzzing and an oscillating sound. If the person is addicted to opiates, it is around the one to one and half-hour mark that their withdrawal symptoms will cease. It is also around this time that people report seeing objects appear to vibrate intensely.

By this time, around the two-hour mark, the full effects of the Ibogaine are at work. This includes hallucinations like color and visual acuity enhancement and distortions such as melting, breathing, morphing, flowing, and tracers. Specifically, the tracer effect is reported to be more intense and more consistent than with any other commonly used psychedelic. Along with visual hallucinations, people also report auditory hallucinations, but these are not the most impactful or important effects.

The most impactful important effects will happen internally.

People report experiencing feelings of catharsis, conceptual or at times delusional thinking, dream potentiation, emotion enhancement, increased libido, increased music appreciation, ego death, mindfulness, novelty enhancement, personal bias suppression, feeling childlike, time distortions, and a feeling rejuvenation.  Although this rejuvenation feeling may take two or three  good nights' rest before it fully presents itself, people report experiencing stimulation for up to 20 hours, making sleep difficult.

# TRADITIONAL USES OF IBOGA

Traditionally iboga was prepared by making fine scrapings of the root bark, breaking it down as much as possible, which could be chewed raw, but often was prepared along with cane juice or sugar, palm wine, or milk. Hunters would take this preparation in low doses as it, reduces sleep, making it possible to resist hunger and fatigue, activates circulation and respiration, and promotes activity. While this is the most common use of the plant in the area, practitioners of Bwiti also use high doses in their rites and rituals.

In high doses, ibogaine produces hallucinatory inebriation that opens the practitioners up to visions that permit contact with ancestors and gods. Due to the fact that when someone uses iboga, they experience a lack of motor coordination and sometimes a state of lethargy lasting four to five days, there is no cultural history for the recreational use of this plant.

# THE BWITI (RELIGION OF EBOGA) CEREMONY

◆ ◆ ◆

### Location

Traditionally in the Bwiti Religion, there is a temple in each village called a Mbandja. This place serves as the location for celebrations, and on occasion, feasts, and initiations. It is where funeral dances are held following the death of a prominent person. The temple may also serve as a meeting room, a courthouse, or a guardhouse if need be.

The Mbandja is a vast rectangular hut, measuring on average 65 feet long and 32 feet wide, that is entirely enclosed in the back. Usually, the sides of the temple are partially closed with a wide opening in the front. The long axis is laid out northeast by southwest, parallel to the route followed by The Fang group during its migration in the last century. (Historians theorize that this move was made to escape slavery and the wars of West Africa and sub-Saharan Africa (9).) The roof is covered with ordinary matting or raphia leaves or, ideally, with leaves of sclerosperma, a sort of dwarf palm. The curved canopy must always be made of sclerosperma leaves. Different columns support the framework of the temple. The great column has a highly sculpted base in which houses the remains of ancestors (mostly skulls and tibias), and is situated at the entrance to the temple, thereby holding great significance.

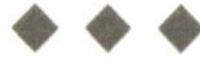

## The Ceremony

*"The subject under the influence of iboga at its peak feels "as if transported by the wind" to the beyond before the house of Christ and God. He is guided to that place by the ancestors, to the sound of the harp."*

- GOLLNHOFER AND SILLANS 1985

For four days, from Wednesday to Sunday, practitioners will only eat Iboga and sip on iboga elixir or water. Wednesday is the first day of the iboga ceremony when people are given Iboga. The ceremony usually begins with a slow procession single file into the temple, and after a short greeting, everyone sits around the edge of the temple. Those in the group taking iboga usually have their faces stained with white powder. The ceremony begins with ritual music played on drums and string instruments. As the speed and volume of the music reach a crescendo, the first dose of Iboga is dispensed by either the priest or priestess. Surprisingly, even babies, newborns, and dogs are given tiny amounts.

On the following day, Thursday, participants prepare for their journey. First red and white designs are marked on the faces of those leading the ceremony. Next, a small fire is created by the river. This is for each participant to sit over while draped in cloth, building a mini sweat lodge designed to help participants sweat out impurities. They are then cleaned in the river.

Friday is the day of sacrifice. Practitioners are placed in a mock grave just outside the temple. Once settled, a chicken is sacrificed in honor of each person, whose blood is then sprinkled over the participants by the Priest or Priestess. They are then covered in sclerosperma leaves. This is done to bury the participant's problems, issues, and illnesses, helping to cleanse further, and purify.

On Saturday, people dress in white, and participants speak their first words since the ceremony began. It is at this time that the priest or priestess will go around to those who are sick and suffering from illness as they are connected at this time to the ancestors and the gods. It is during this time that priests and priestesses can diagnose and cure people. This is the most individualized part of the ceremony where certain spells, incantations, or traditional healing methods are applied. At this time, the music comes to a halt. At the end of the ritual initiation on Sunday morning, you have your first meal, and are reborn.

# MODERN USE OF IBOGA AND IBOGAINE

In the west, iboga, and therefore ibogaine, have had little to no cultural history, and both mainly went unknown and unrecognized by science for decades. No one in the west had ever thought of using ibogaine except as an anti-fatigue medication, and its use was almost exclusive to France and French colonies. After all, it was the Frenchmen that wrote the first papers on ibogaine. Although noteworthy, the current interest in ibogaine and its anti-addictive properties far outweigh the societal good and usefulness.

Modern ibogaine ceremonies should be carried out with some level of medical oversight. If not under the direct supervision of a doctor, people wishing to do ibogaine therapy should still have a medical check-up before treatment as there are some very real cardiological issues. A small percentage of people with a specific heart condition, called a prolonged QT rhythm, can put them at high risk for having a severe negative cardiologic issue that, if not treated immediately, can lead to cardiac arrest, and even death. Other potential complications can arise from the use of SSRI or

MAOI medications, having a history of mania (as this sacrament can precipitate manic symptoms), or having active panic attacks.

Once a person is cleared before the ceremony begins, usually a few other recommendations are made to participants. This is to avoid alcohol or any psychoactive substances at least two to three days before the iboga ceremony. The longer, the better. For those using ibogaine to treat opiate addiction, it is highly recommended to wait to begin until the participant is experiencing full withdrawal. This can range from as few as eight hours for drugs like heroin, and up to three days for methadone. Another recommendation is to set an intention.All retreats will say Meditation and intention are essential to get the most from experience.

When attending one of the more traditional style retreats they will bethat are modeled after the Bwiti ceremonies. According to one retreat, "Each Iboga ceremony starts around a fire. This is an important part of honoring sacred Bwiti tradition."(11). This is followed by a fireside talk where they "impart vital wisdom… (with topics surrounding) connecting to our soul, loving ourselves, overriding the ego, empowering ourselves, finding inner peace."(11). Bwiti music will be an integral part of the ceremony as it is believed to help with connection and can serve to enhance the experience. The retreat goes on to detail the rest of the process, " The journey continues throughout the evening and into the following morning. After dawn breaks, guests are invited to return to their rooms… (beginning) a day of rest and discovery. This entire day is about introspection and typically is spent with no sleep, reviewing the messages and teachings we have received from Iboga."(11) Often, this integration period is most important to maximize the benefits of the treatment.

According the Iboga Tree Healing House, a company offering medically supervised ibogaine retreats state that their treatments usually follow this rhythm. Patients are evaluated on the first day of arrival to ensure that ibogaine will be safe. The next day, "We usually start your ibogaine treatment in the morning."(12). They note, "For addicts... between 30min to 2 hours after ibogaine administration, you will start to feel a bit different and notice that the usual withdrawal symptoms are gone."(12). After taking ibogaine, patients will lay down comfortably in a darkened room.

At the ready is a therapist who can help deal with any challenging emotions and act to reassure the patient if they have an intense experience. The company goes on to say that at " approx. 3-4 hours... people still experience visions, although they are less intense, and you gradually shift towards more meditative, introspective states. There is now time to evaluate the visionary experiences"(12).  During the final stage of the treatment, when the effects begin to wane, they "play softening music which eventually leads you to a well-deserved sleep."(12) They go on to mention, "You should note that ibogaine prevents you from sleeping, so it may take many hours for you to fall asleep."(12) Most patients report feeling awake, rested, and hungry after a good sleep. It is highly recommended that all who go to an ibogaine ceremony attend an after-care program for 6-12 months as this will result in the best outcome.

# AN ANCIENT TOOL FOR A MODERN PROBLEM

The modern world has come with many benefits to lots of people. From better healthcare that has led to an increase in life expectancy to a modern logistics system that has allowed global trade, there are countless examples of how life has improved with time. Despite the constant advances, there seems to be one global issue that seems to be getting worse, the issue of both behavioral and pharmacological addiction.

From alcoholism to opiates and porn to phones, there seem to be ever-increasing rates of self-reporting and admissions for treatment. Despite having come this far, the options for treating these behaviors come down to a few strategies. Replacement, things like methadone and the nicotine patch that substitute the more harmful behavior with something less destructive. Deterrence such as lengthy prison sentences in the hopes that this will keep people from behaving a certain way. And/or therapy which seeks to modify behavioral patterns and keep people from acting on addictive impulses. Unfortunately, this system has been proven to be less than effective in many cases leaving people to suffer through the meat grinder that addiction is.

It is this need for a new solution in the area of addiction treatment that is driving the intrest in alternative medications,especially into ibogaine and iboga for the multiple ways that it is proving to be beneficial in the fight against addiction. Looking at the work of Lotsof and the first studies of ibogaine it was clear this would be a game changer. The efficacy of ibogaine in different groups suffering from addiction(4,5,6,7) has up to this point remained unmatched. Although other psychedelics are definitely benifical and hold their own when it comes to psychedelic therapy.

Ibogaine's extraordinary pharmacological profile makes it a groundbreaking contender in the fight against addiction! Its powerful dissociative and psychedelic effects, combined with the cascade of diverse neurotransmitters, hold incredible promise for reducing cravings and alleviating withdrawal symptoms. The potential for promoting neuroplasticity and fostering holistic healing offers a refreshing and transformative approach to recovery. While we have encouraging anecdotal evidence, the call for more research and careful clinical application is vital to unlock its full potential safely. The future of addiction treatment could be brighter than ever with ibogaine in the spotlight! Ibogaine is linked to some truly amazing 3 to 6 month outcomes(11,12).

If a person has tried several treatment options without success, is in good health, and has access to a safe and controlled environment, they should have the option to consider ibogaine therapy, which has repeatedly demonstrated its effectiveness.

23

# ACKNOWLEDGEMENT


1.    Dybowski J, Landrin E (1901). "PLANT CHEMISTRY. Concerning Iboga, its excitement-producing properties, its composition, and the new alkaloid it contains, ibogaine". Comptes rendus de l'Académie des Sciences Vol 133

2.    Dzoljic ED, Kaplan CD, Dzoljic MR.(1998) Effect of ibogaine on naloxone-precipitated withdrawal syndrome in chronic morphine-dependent rats. Archives Internationales de Pharmacodynamie et de Therapie.

3.    Aubry-Lecomte, Charles Eugène(1864) Note sur quelque poisons de la côte occidentale d'Afrique. Revue Maritime et Coloniale, vol. XII,.

4.    Lotsof, H.S. 1989. U.S. Patent No. 4,857,523.

5.    Lotsof, H.S. 1986. U.S. Patent No. 4,587,243.

6.    Lotsof, H.S. 1985. U.S. Patent No. 4,499,096.

7.    Lotsof, H.S. 1991. U.S. Patent No. 5,026,697.

8.    Popik P, Skolnick P (1998). Pharmacology of Ibogaine and Ibogaine-Related Alkaloids. The Alkaloids: Chemistry and Biology. Vol. 52. Academic Press. pp. 197–231

9.    Anthony Appiah; Henry Louis Gates (2010). Encyclopedia of Africa. Oxford University Press. pp. 415–419

10.    Dhahir, H.I. 1971. A comparative study on the toxicity of ibogaine and serotonin. Thesis, Ph.D. In Toxicology, Indiana University

11.  Awaken Your Soul. Ibogaine Treatment center

12.  Iboga Tree Healing Center. Ibogaine treatment center

# BOOKS BY THIS AUTHOR

## Amphetamine Addiction: The Amphetamine Epidemic

"The Amphetamine Epidemic" provides a comprehensive and in-depth examination of one of the most pressing public health crises of the 21st century. This book delves into the rise, spread, and devastating impact of amphetamine use and abuse, shedding light on the social, economic, and medical implications of this global phenomenon.

Part I: The Rise of Amphetamines The book traces the origins of amphetamines, which were first synthesized in the late 19th century, and their gradual integration into various medical treatments and military use during World War II. As the pharmaceutical industry evolved, so did the availability and accessibility of amphetamines, leading to their widespread prescription for medical conditions like attention deficit hyperactivity disorder (ADHD) and narcolepsy.

As prescription rates skyrocketed, the unintended consequences of overprescribing and diversion began to surface. Readers will explore the alarming escalation of amphetamine abuse and the development of illegal manufacturing and distribution networks. Moreover, the book examines the societal impact, including the strain on healthcare systems, the criminal justice system, and the overall economic burden.

## Cerebrolysin: The Next Evolution Of Medicine

Cerebrolysin is a captivating and informative book that explores the fascinating world of Cerebrolysin, a unique and revolutionary neurotrophic agent. Written using the most up-to-date scientific research, this book delves into the remarkable properties and potential applications of Cerebrolysin in enhancing brain function and improving cognitive abilities.

The story begins with an introduction to Cerebrolysin, a peptide-based drug derived from porcine brain tissue, which has gained significant attention in the scientific community. With its ability to stimulate neuronal growth, enhance synaptic connectivity, and modulate neurotransmitter activity, Cerebrolysin has emerged as a promising tool for treating various neurological conditions and optimizing brain performance.

Read along as the book explores the intricate mechanisms through which Cerebrolysin interacts with the brain, shedding light on the fascinating interplay between neurobiology and cognitive enhancement.

Furthermore, the book explores the potential future applications of Cerebrolysin, including its role in neurorehabilitation, cognitive enhancement in healthy individuals, and its influence on the aging brain. The authors also address important considerations surrounding the use of Cerebrolysin and delve into ongoing research, discussing potential risks and challenges associated with its implementation.

Hopefully I have managed to engages readers of all types with its blend of scientific insights, compelling narratives, and a vision for a future where Cerebrolysin plays a significant role in unlocking the full potential of the human mind.

## Drug Withdrawal: The Science Of Healing Your Body

An insightful and compassionate recovery book that offers a guiding light to individuals and families seeking healing and empowerment on their path to recovery. With a blend of personal anecdotes, expert advice, and practical tools, this book serves as a trustworthy companion for anyone facing various challenges, be it addiction, mental health struggles, trauma, or other forms of adversity.

Author KM Schaeffer, a person in long-term recovery brings a unique perspective to this book. Combining professional expertise with personal experiences, he offer a compassionate and relatable voice that resonates with readers at a profound level. The book speaks directly to the readers' hearts, acknowledging their pain while offering hope and inspiration for a brighter future.

## Happy And Healthy: Tips And Tricks For A Better Life

a world where chaos and uncertainty seem to dominate, "Happy and Healthy" serves as a compassionate guide for navigating life's most challenging moments. This book is a roadmap to emotional healing, self-awareness, and personal growth, offering powerful tools to help you rise above the turmoil and discover peace and meaning. Through ten transformative chapters, you'll explore essential strategies to care for your mind, body, and soul, with practical insights and actionable steps that can bring immediate relief.

# ABOUT THE AUTHOR

## Km Schaeffer

KM Schaeffer is an author and researcher deeply passionate about the intersections of neuroscience, addiction recovery, and alternative medicine. With a focus on exploring innovative therapies, Schaeffer's work delves into the healing potential of substances like ibogaine, cerebrolysin, and other cutting-edge treatments. His writings aim to empower individuals struggling with addiction, mental health challenges, and cognitive decline by providing them with practical insights and scientifically-backed solutions. Through his books, Schaeffer offers a compassionate and well-researched approach, making complex topics accessible to readers seeking hope, healing, and personal transformation.